# Gut Health Revolution

The Benefits of Vital Biome Gut Health 4-in-1 Supplements for Men and Women

Hazel Knight

# Copyright © 2024 by Hazel Knight

# Contents

# Chapter 1: Introduction

## My Experience with Vital Biome Gut Health 4-in-1

A few years ago, I started taking Vital Biome Gut Health 4-in-1 supplements because I was having recurring digestive problems. I was now accustomed to having bloating, inconsistent bowel movements, and general abdominal discomfort. Nothing that I tried, including changing my diet and using over-the-counter medications, appeared to offer long-lasting comfort.

Desperate to find a remedy, I began reading up on gut health and discovered the notion of the gut microbiome. I was intrigued by the possibility that an imbalance in my digestive tract could be the cause of my stomach problems. This is how I came across the Vital Biome Gut Health 4-in-1 supplements, which included probiotics, prebiotics, digestive enzymes, and fiber to improve digestive health.

I decided to test these vitamins despite my skepticism. It was difficult in the beginning days as my body got used to the new routine. Even though I had some alterations in my bowel movements and some mild bloating, I was determined to persevere. I started to see little gains over time. My digestion seemed more regular and effective, and the constant bloating began to fade.

The changes become increasingly noticeable after a few weeks. For the first time in a long time, I felt lighter, more energized, and less prone to intestinal problems.

The biggest adjustment was the enhancement of my general well-being. I noticed that I had more regular energy levels and that I felt tired less often. I later found that this could be attributed to the gut-brain axis, a fascinating relationship between gut health and mental health. Even my mood seemed more consistent.

Inspired by these encouraging developments, I maintained my Vital Biome Gut Health 4-in-1 vitamin regimen. With time, the advantages went beyond digestive well-being. My immune system seemed to be functioning better because I saw a decrease in infections and colds. I also looked to be in better health overall, which was reflected in my skin.

In addition to improving my digestive health, this experience ignited a love for learning about the gut's vital function in general health. My success with Vital Biome Gut Health 4-in-1 supplements motivated me to share my story with others who may be having similar issues. With this book, I hope you will be able to learn about the many advantages of supporting gut health and start down your path to wellness.

## The Significance of Gut Health

Gut health has recently emerged as an important aspect of overall wellness. The gut, commonly known as the "second brain," is essential for digestion, immunological function, mental health, and chronic disease prevention.

Understanding and maintaining gut health is critical for a lively and healthy lifestyle.

The gut microbiome is made up of billions of microorganisms such as bacteria, viruses, and fungi. These little residents are not passive dwellers; they actively contribute to our health in a variety of ways.

They aid digestion, create critical nutrients, guard against infections, and control our immune system. Dysbiosis, or an imbalance in the gut microbiome, can cause a variety of health problems, including digestive troubles, autoimmune illnesses, mental health disorders, and obesity.

## Overview of Vital Biome Gut Health 4-in-1 Supplements.

The Vital Biome Gut Health 4-in-1 supplement supports and improves gut health by combining four vital ingredients: probiotics, prebiotics, digestive enzymes, and fiber. Each of these nutrients has a distinct and important purpose in keeping a healthy digestive tract.

- **Probiotics:** These helpful bacteria assist to balance the gut microbiome, enhance digestion, and strengthen the immune system.

- **Prebiotics:** Non-digestible fibers that nourish the gut's beneficial bacteria, encouraging their development and activity.

- **Digestive Enzymes** are proteins that aid in the breakdown of food into nutrients that the body can absorb, hence aiding digestion and nutritional absorption.

- **Fiber** is necessary for regulating bowel motions, avoiding constipation, and maintaining overall gut health.

The advantages of every one of these components will be thoroughly discussed in this book, along with helpful tips on how to use the Vital Biome Gut Health 4-in-1 supplement in your daily routine to achieve maximum health.

## Purpose and Scope of the Book

The major purpose of this book is to give a complete approach to understanding and enhancing gut health with the Vital Biome Gut Health 4-in-1 supplement. Whether you're new to the notion of gut health or want to expand your understanding, this book provides essential insights and practical advice to help you on your path.

We will discuss the science of gut health, explain how the components of the Vital Biome Gut Health 4-in-1 supplement operate, and offer step-by-step instructions for utilizing these supplements properly. Furthermore, we will look at nutritional and lifestyle adjustments that might help your gut health.

By the end of this book, you will have a complete grasp of the significance of gut health, the advantages of the Vital Biome Gut Health 4-in-1 supplement, and how to take proactive actions to enhance your digestive health and general quality of life.

# Chapter 2: Understanding Gut Health

## The Overview of the Gut Microbiome

Our digestive system is home to a diverse collection of bacteria called the gut microbiome. This ecosystem comprises bacteria, viruses, fungi, and other microorganisms essential to preserving health and averting illness. Proper gut function and general health depend on the diversity and balance of these microbes.

**Composition and Functionality**

1. Bacteria: The most researched element of the microbiome, gut bacteria are necessary for immune system regulation, vitamin production (including B12 and K), and food digestion. Actinobacteria, Proteobacteria, Bacteroidetes, and Firmicutes are important bacterial groups.

2. Viruses: Despite being frequently linked to illness, a large number of gut-dwelling viruses, known as bacteriophages, particularly infect bacteria and aid in the preservation of bacterial balance.

3. Fungi: In the stomach, yeasts and molds aid in the absorption of nutrients and the development of immunological responses. The most well-known fungi in the stomach are species of Candida.

4. Archaea and Other Microorganisms: These less well-known microorganisms are important for digestion and health because they produce methane and cycle nutrients.

## Key Functions

- Digestion and Metabolism: Microbes help absorb nutrients and create energy by breaking down carbohydrates, fibers, and proteins.

- Immune System Regulation: The gut microbiome protects against infections and moderates the immune system, reducing hyperactive reactions that might trigger autoimmune disorders.

- Barrier Function: The gut lining serves as a barrier to keep dangerous chemicals out of the bloodstream, and it is maintained by beneficial bacteria.

- Neurotransmitter Production: The gut-brain link is strengthened by the production of neurotransmitters like serotonin, which affect mood and mental health.

# The Effects of Gut Health on Overall Well-Being

The impact of the gut microbiome goes well beyond digesting. This is how it affects different areas of health:

1. Immune Function: The stomach contains around 70% of the immune system. A well-balanced microbiome lowers the risk of inflammatory disorders and aids in infection defense.

2. Mental Health: Given that the stomach and the brain communicate in both directions through the gut-brain axis, gut health has a major impact on mental health. Gut bacteria imbalances have been linked to anxiety, depression, and other mental health conditions.

3. Weight Management: The control of appetite, fat storage, and metabolism are all impacted by the bacteria in the gut. While some bacterial profiles support leanness, others are linked to fat.

4. Chronic Diseases: Dysbiosis has been connected to several chronic illnesses, such as inflammatory bowel disease (IBD), diabetes, and cardiovascular disease.

5. Skin Health: By lowering inflammation and restoring equilibrium to the skin microbiome, a healthy stomach can help promote cleaner skin.

## Common Gut Health Problems

1. Dysbiosis: An imbalance in the microbiome of the gut, frequently brought on by disease, stress, antibiotic usage, or

a bad diet. Constipation, diarrhea, gas, and bloating are among the symptoms.

2. Leaky Gut Syndrome: Bacteria and poisons can enter the circulation through increased intestinal permeability, causing inflammation and perhaps exacerbating autoimmune disorders.

3. Irritable Bowel Syndrome (IBS): Symptoms of this functional gastrointestinal condition include bloating, changed bowel habits, and abdominal discomfort.

4. Inflammatory Bowel Disease (IBD): Consists of ailments involving persistent inflammation of the digestive system, such as ulcerative colitis and Crohn's disease.

5. Small Intestinal Bacterial Overgrowth (SIBO): Symptoms such as gas, bloating, and malabsorption are caused by an overgrowth of bacteria in the small intestine.

To improve gut health, one must first understand these problems. We will examine the elements of the Vital Biome Gut Health 4-in-1 supplement and how they solve these typical gut health issues in the upcoming chapter.

# Chapter 3: Components of Vital Biome Gut Health 4-in-1 Supplements

We will go into great detail about each of the Vital Biome Gut Health 4-in-1 supplements' components in this chapter. Probiotics, prebiotics, digestive enzymes, and fiber work synergistically to maintain and improve gut health in these supplements.

## Probiotics: The Good Bacteria

Probiotics are live microorganisms that give the host health advantages when taken in sufficient doses. They are mostly made up of healthy bacterial strains and certain yeasts that support the upkeep of a balanced gut microbiome.

### Advantages of Probiotics

1. Restoring Microbial Balance: Probiotics have the potential to assist in the restoration and sustenance of a normal gut microbiome balance, particularly following disturbances caused by antibiotic usage.

2. Improved Digestion: Some probiotic strains help break down lactose and fiber, which enhances overall digestion and lessens bloating and gas sensations.

3. Immune Support: Probiotics improve the function of the gut barrier and promote the synthesis of chemicals that regulate the immune system, which helps to maintain immunological health.

4. Anti-inflammatory Effects: Certain probiotics generate short-chain fatty acids (SCFAs), which support gut health and have anti-inflammatory qualities.

5. Mental Health Benefits: A new study indicates that probiotics may affect the gut-brain axis and help reduce feelings of depression and anxiety.

**Common Probiotic Strains**

- Lactobacillus: Known for aiding with digestion and immune support, this bacterium is present in yogurt and fermented foods.

- Bifidobacterium: Found primarily in the colon, this bacteria aids in the production of vitamins and the breakdown of dietary fiber.

- Saccharomyces boulardii: A healthy yeast that improves digestive health and may help avoid diarrhea caused by antibiotics or infections.

# Prebiotics: Feeding the Healthy Bacteria

Prebiotics are indigestible fibers that provide nourishment to probiotics and other advantageous microorganisms in the gastrointestinal tract. They make it to the colon, where bacteria ferment them, after passing through the digestive system undigested.

## Advantages of Prebiotics

1. Promoting Gut Health: Prebiotics promote the growth and activity of beneficial bacteria such as bifidobacteria and lactobacilli, which increase gut microbial diversity.

2. Improving Digestive Function: Prebiotics support regular bowel movements and lessen constipation symptoms by encouraging the growth of good bacteria.

3. Improving Mineral Absorption: Prebiotics may help the body absorb minerals like magnesium and calcium, which are good for the health of the bones.

4. Supporting immunological Function: Prebiotics, like probiotics, aid in bolstering the intestinal barrier and bolstering immunological responses, which may lower the risk of infection.

5. Potential Benefits for Weight Management: Research indicates that prebiotics may affect the appetite and satiety hormones, which may help with weight management.

**Common Sources of Prebiotics**

- Inulin: Located in food variety of vegetables, herbs, and fruits such as bananas, garlic, onions, leeks, asparagus, and artichokes.

- Fructooligosaccharides (FOS): Naturally present in fruits and vegetables such as asparagus, leeks, and Jerusalem artichokes.

- Galactooligosaccharides (GOS): Found in several dairy products and legumes (beans, lentils).

## Digestive Enzymes: Boosting Metabolism

Specialized proteins called digestive enzymes reduce large food molecules into smaller, more absorbable components that the body can utilize.

**Types of Digestive Enzymes**

1. Amylases: Convert carbohydrates into glucose and other simple sugars.

2. Proteases: Break down proteins to produce amino acids.

3. Lipases: Produce glycerol and fatty acids from fats.

4. Cellulases: Produce glucose by breaking down cellulose (fiber).

5. Lactases: Break down milk sugar, and lactose, into glucose and galactose.

## Advantages of Digestive Enzymes

- Enhanced Absorption of Nutrients: Digestion enzymes facilitate better absorption of nutrients by dissolving food into smaller molecules, which is particularly beneficial for people with digestive issues or enzyme deficiencies.

- Reduced Digestive Discomfort: By assisting in the digestion of particular nutrients, enzyme supplements can help reduce symptoms like indigestion, gas, and bloating.

- Support for Digestive Disorders: By enhancing digestive efficiency, they may help people with ailments like lactose intolerance, pancreatic insufficiency, or IBS.

# Fiber: Digestive Health's Unsung Hero

Plant-based foods contain fiber, a kind of carbohydrate that the body is unable to absorb or digest. It remains intact as it moves through the digestive system and offers several health advantages.

## Types and Advantages of Fiber

1. Soluble Fiber: This fiber dissolves in water to produce a gel-like substance that can control blood sugar and cholesterol.

2. Insoluble Fiber: Promotes regular bowel movements and prevents constipation by adding bulk to stool and refusing to dissolve in water.

3. Prebiotic Fiber: Promotes the growth and activity of good gut bacteria by acting as food for them.

## Sources of Fiber

- Vegetables and Fruits: Broccoli, carrots, spinach, apples, and berries.

- Whole Grains: Brown rice, whole wheat, quinoa, and oats.

- Legumes: Peas, beans, lentils, and chickpeas.

- Nuts and Seeds: Pumpkin, flax, chia, and almond seeds.

# Chapter 4: How to use Vital Biome Gut Health 4-in-1 Supplements

Understanding and optimizing the benefits of Vital Biome Gut Health 4-in-1 supplements is essential for effectively incorporating them into your routine. Here's a detailed guide to using these nutritional supplements to improve your digestive health:

## Choosing the Right Supplement:

When choosing Vital Biome Gut Health 4-in-1 supplements, examine the formulation that best suits your lifestyle and interests. These supplements are available in a variety of formats, including capsules, powders, and chewables. Choose a form that is handy and easy to integrate into your everyday routine.

Make sure the supplement you purchase contains high-quality nutrients including probiotics, prebiotics, digestive enzymes, and a combination of soluble and insoluble fiber. Quality is essential for getting the full range of benefits these supplements provide.

## Recommended dosage and timing:

To reap the full advantages of Vital Biome Gut Health 4-in-1 supplements, follow the manufacturer's recommended dosage instructions or consult your healthcare physician. Dosages vary depending on the substance and its intended purpose. Typically, supplements are taken once or twice a day with meals to aid digestion and nutritional absorption.

- Probiotics: Take probiotic supplements with your meals to help digestion. When probiotics are consumed with food, the live bacteria survive better in the stomach's acidic environment.

- Prebiotics: These can be taken at any time of day, but are most effective with fiber-rich meals. Prebiotics nurture probiotics and other healthy microorganisms in the gut.

- Digestive Enzymes: Digestive enzyme supplements are typically taken with meals to aid in the breakdown of food into absorbable nutrients. To achieve the best effects, follow the precise recommendations on the supplement packaging.

- Fiber: Make sure you get enough fiber throughout the day, whether from whole meals or supplements. Fiber supplements can be taken with plenty of water to promote bowel regularity and digestive health.

## Integrating Supplements into Your Routine:

Consistency is essential when taking Vital Biome Gut Health 4-in-1 supplements. To create a habit, incorporate them into your daily routine at the same time every day.

This consistency ensures that you continue to benefit from improved digestion, immunological function, and overall well-being.

## Extra Tips for Usage:

- Monitor Effects: Pay attention to how your body reacts to the supplements. Observe any changes in digestion, bowel motions, or overall health.

- Adjust as Needed: Depending on your specific requirements and response, you may need to change the dosage or timing of your supplements. If you have any specific concerns or queries, consult a healthcare professional.

- Combine with Healthy Habits: Supplements are most effective when coupled with a well-balanced diet high in fruits, vegetables, whole grains, and lean proteins. Drinking enough water and engaging in regular exercise promotes digestive health.

Understanding the components of Vital Biome Gut Health 4-in-1 supplements and how to utilize them successfully will help you improve your digestive health and general well-being.

Consistent use, combined with good living practices, boosts the advantages of probiotics, prebiotics, digestive enzymes, and fiber, resulting in a more balanced gut microbiome and improved digestion.

# Chapter 5: Practical Tips for Optimal Gut Health

Maintaining good gut health entails more than just taking supplements; it requires a balanced approach to nutrition and lifestyle. Here are some practical recommendations for supporting your gut health and getting the most out of Vital Biome Gut Health 4-in-1 supplements:

**1. Adopt a Fiber-Rich Diet:**

- Incorporate Whole Foods: Incorporate plenty of fruits, vegetables, whole grains, legumes, nuts, and seeds into your diet. These meals include important nutrients and fiber, which nurture good gut bacteria and promote digestive regularity.

- Variety matters: Aim for a variety of fiber sources to promote a healthy gut microbiome. Different forms of fiber feed different bacteria in the stomach, which helps to maintain microbial diversity and health.

## 2. Focus on Probiotic-Rich Foods:

- Include Fermented Foods: Yogurt, kefir, sauerkraut, kimchi, and kombucha are high in natural probiotics. Regular eating of these foods complements probiotic pills by offering a diverse range of living microorganisms that promote intestinal health.

- Select Quality: Choose fermented foods that include living and active cultures, as fermentation increases the availability of beneficial bacteria.

## 3. Limit Sugar and Processed Foods:

- Prevent Excess Sugar: High-sugar diets can upset the balance of gut bacteria, causing inflammation and digestive difficulties. Reduce your intake of sugary snacks, sweets, and beverages.

- Minimize Processed Foods: Processed meals frequently contain chemicals and preservatives, which can harm gut health. Choose complete, unprocessed foods wherever possible to promote a healthy gut microbiome.

## 4. Stay Hydrated:

- Drink Lots of Water: Adequate hydration is crucial for good digestion and general health. Water softens feces and facilitates food flow through the digestive tract, thus reducing constipation.

## 5. Effective Stress Management:

- Use Stress-Relieving Techniques: Chronic stress can impair gut health by influencing gut motility and bacteria composition. To boost general well-being, use stress-relieving methods such as yoga, meditation, deep breathing exercises, or outdoor activities.

## 6. Regular exercise promotes digestive health.

- Physical activity promotes regular bowel movements and maintains a healthy gut microbiome. Aim for at least 30 minutes of moderate-intensity exercise on most days of the week to improve digestive function and general health.

## 7. Ensure Adequate Sleep:

- Prioritize Quality Sleep: Lack of sleep can harm gut health by altering the gut microbiome and raising inflammation. Aim for 7-9 hours of quality sleep per night to promote good digestion and general health.

## 8. Seek additional support:

- Speak with a healthcare professional: If you have specific digestive issues or health conditions, speak with your doctor or a trained nutritionist. They can offer personalized recommendations and advice on how to improve your gut health.

Incorporating these practical strategies into your daily routine, along with Vital Biome Gut Health 4-in-1 vitamins, will help you support your digestive health and general well-being. A balanced diet, regular physical activity, enough hydration, stress management, quality sleep, and appropriate nutrition all work together to promote good gut health.

# Chapter 6: Common Misconceptions about Gut Health

Gut health is becoming increasingly popular, yet it is typically surrounded by myths and misconceptions. In this chapter, we'll debunk some common beliefs and provide facts based on research to help you make educated choices regarding your digestive health.

**Myth 1: All Bacteria Are Harmful.**

**Reality:** Not all bacteria are harmful. Our bodies contain billions of helpful bacteria, particularly in the gut. These microorganisms are necessary for digestion, nutrition absorption, and immunological function. Probiotics, or "good" bacteria found in supplements and fermented foods, serve to maintain a healthy balance in the gut microbiome, which is essential for general health.

**Myth 2: Probiotics Alone Can Treat All Digestive Problems**

**Reality:** Probiotics are useful, but they are not a cure-all. They function best when accompanied by a nutritious diet high in prebiotics (fibers that feed good bacteria), enough hydration, and other lifestyle variables including regular exercise and stress management. Probiotics are part of a comprehensive approach to gut health, not a stand-alone treatment.

## Myth 3: Fiber is only necessary if you have constipation

**Reality:** Fiber is beneficial to everyone, not just those with constipation. Dietary fiber promotes regular bowel movements, blood sugar regulation, cholesterol reduction, and a healthy gut microbiome. Both soluble and insoluble fibers are necessary for good digestive function.

## Myth 4: Gut Health Supplements Work Instantly.

**Reality:** Gut health supplements, such as Vital Biome Gut Health 4-in-1, might take some time to show results. It may take several weeks of constant use to notice improvements in digestion, immunological function, and overall health. Patience and persistence are essential while using these supplements.

## Myth 5: More probiotics equals better results

**Reality:** When it comes to probiotics, more doesn't always mean better. The efficiency of probiotics is determined by the individual strains utilized and their capacity to survive the digestive process. Quality and the optimal strain mix are more essential than quantity. It's also critical to adhere to the specified dosage on the supplement package.

## Myth 6: Gut Health Only Impacts Digestion

**Reality:** Gut health has far-reaching impacts that go beyond digesting. A healthy gut microbiome affects the immune system, mental health, skin health, and even weight control. The gut-brain axis, for example, demonstrates the link between gut health and mental well-being, which influences mood and cognitive performance.

## Myth 7: Prebiotics and Probiotics Are Identical

**Reality:** Prebiotics and probiotics are distinct, yet complimentary. Probiotics are living beneficial bacteria, whereas prebiotics are indigestible carbohydrates that nourish these bacteria. Both are important for a healthy gut microbiome and should be part of a well-balanced diet.

## Myth 8: If you eat healthy, you don't need supplements.

**Reality:** While a good diet is essential for gut health, supplements can help when food consumption is insufficient or when certain health conditions impair nutrient absorption. Vital Biome Gut Health 4-in-1 supplements can help cover nutritional shortages and improve overall gut health.

Understanding the reality of gut health enables you to make more informed decisions and avoid common myths. Gut health is multidimensional and includes nutrition, lifestyle, and supplements. By refuting these misconceptions, we might adopt a more enlightened and successful approach to gut health.

# Chapter 7: Scientific Backing and Research for Vital Biome Gut Health 4-in-1 Supplements

When it comes to establishing the efficacy of supplements and the components that make them up, scientific research is an extremely important factor. The purpose of this chapter is to explore the scientific data that supports the utilization of digestive enzymes, fiber, probiotics, and prebiotics, which are the primary components of the Vital Biome Gut Health 4-in-1 supplements.

## 1. Probiotics.

The consumption of sufficient quantities of probiotics, which are living bacteria, has been shown to provide health advantages. It is well-documented in the scientific literature that probiotics provide significant health advantages.

## Key Studies and Findings:

- Gut Health and Digestive Support: A comprehensive analysis published in the journal Nutrients indicates that probiotics can help improve symptoms of irritable bowel syndrome (IBS), including bloating, gas, and abdominal pain.

- Enhancement of the Immune System: It was discovered in a study that was published in Frontiers in Immunology that probiotics have the power to impact the immune system, which in turn increases its capacity to fight infections and reduce inflammation.

- Mental Health: According to research published in **Psychiatry Research,** probiotics can improve mental health by affecting the gut-brain axis and lowering symptoms of depression and anxiety.

## 2. Prebiotics

Prebiotics are non-digestible fibers that serve as food for helpful gut bacteria. They encourage the growth and activity of these bacteria, supporting overall gut health.

## Key Studies and Findings:

- Gut Microbiome Support: An article in **The Journal of Nutrition** states that prebiotics stimulate the growth of beneficial bacteria, enhancing gut health and function.

- Digestive Health: Research in **Alimentary Pharmacology & Therapeutics** reveals that prebiotics can enhance bowel regularity and lessen symptoms of constipation.

- Immunological Function: A study in **The British Journal of Nutrition** indicated that prebiotics can increase the immunological response, potentially reducing the occurrence of infections.

## 3. Digestive Enzymes:

Digestive enzymes are proteins that aid the digestion of food into absorbable nutrients. They are needed for healthy digestion and nutritional absorption.

### Key Studies and Findings:

- Digestive Efficiency: Research in the journal **Gastroenterology & Hepatology** reveals that digestive enzyme supplements can increase the digestion and absorption of nutrients, particularly in those with enzyme shortages.

- Symptom Relief for IBS: Research in **The American Journal of Gastroenterology** indicated that digestive enzymes can help lessen symptoms of IBS, such as bloating and gas.

## 4. Fiber

Dietary fiber is vital for supporting good digestion and encouraging regular bowel movements. It also has a part in maintaining a healthy weight and minimizing the risk of chronic diseases.

**Key Studies and Findings:**

- Bowel Regularity: A comprehensive study in **The Journal of the American Medical Association** (JAMA) reveals that dietary fiber can enhance bowel regularity and avoid constipation.

- Weight Management: Research in **The American Journal of Clinical Nutrition** reveals that a high-fiber diet can benefit weight management by enhancing appetite and reducing overall calorie consumption.

- Chronic Disease Prevention: A study published in **Lancet** indicated that higher dietary fiber intake is related to a lower risk of cardiovascular disease, type 2 diabetes, and colorectal cancer.

The scientific data supporting the components of Vital Biome Gut Health 4-in-1 supplements is substantial. Probiotics, prebiotics, digestive enzymes, and fiber each offer well-documented benefits for digestive health, immunological support, mental well-being, and overall health. Incorporating these elements into your health regimen can provide full support for your gut and overall health.

# Chapter 8: Potential Side Effects of Vital Biome Gut Health 4-in-1 Supplements and How to Deal with Them

While the majority of people find Vital Biome Gut Health 4-in-1 supplements to be safe, some people may have adverse effects. Understanding these potential side effects and how to deal with them will allow you to use these supplements more effectively.

## 1. Digestive discomfort

Signs: Initial side effects like bloating, gas, and pain in the abdomen are usual while your body adjusts to the new nutrients.

## Handling Advice:

- Start Slowly: To give your stomach time to adjust, start with a smaller dose and work your way up to the suggested quantity.

- Remain Hydrated: To aid your digestive system in processing the additional fiber and other ingredients, sip on plenty of water.

- Keep an eye on your diet: Make sure your diet is well-balanced and rich in different forms of fiber. This may lessen upset in the digestive system.


## 2. Changes in Bowel Movements

Signs: Changes in bowel movements, such as increased frequency, softer stools, or diarrhea, may occur for certain persons.


## Handling Advice:

- Adjust Fiber Intake: Rather than making abrupt adjustments, gradually increase your intake of fiber. Your digestive system may adjust more easily as a result of this.

- Balance With Soluble Fiber: If you have diarrhea, try eating more soluble fiber (found in oats, apples, and carrots), which can help solidify your stools.

- Speak with a Professional: Seek medical advice if your bowel movements persist and become more severe.


## 3. Hypersensitivity Responses

Signs: Rarely, but possible, some people may experience adverse responses to particular probiotic strains or fiber types in the supplements.

## Handling Advice:

- Read Labels Carefully: Before beginning the supplement, look through the ingredient list for any possible allergies.

- Allergy Test: If you've ever had allergies in the past, you might want to have an allergy test from a medical professional.

- Discontinue Use: If you get symptoms like a rash, itching, swelling, or trouble breathing, stop taking the supplement right once and visit a doctor.

## 4. How Medications Interact

Signs: Certain supplement components may interact with prescription drugs, reducing their effectiveness or producing unfavorable side effects.

## Handling Advice:

- Consult Your Doctor: Before beginning the supplements, let your doctor know if you are taking any drugs, particularly immunosuppressants or antibiotics.

- Monitor Your Health: When you combine supplements with pharmaceuticals, be aware of any changes in your condition or adverse effects and let your healthcare professional know about them.

## 5. Excessive Fiber Consumption

Signs: Constipation, diarrhea, gas, and bloating can result from consuming too much fiber.

## Handling Advice:

- Recommended Dosage: Adhere to the suggested dosage shown on the package of the product. Refrain from exceeding the dosage in the hopes of achieving quicker outcomes.

- Increase Fiber Gradually: Gradually add fiber to your diet so that your body can become used to it.

## 6. Temporary Symptom Increase

Signs: Some people may experience a temporary increase in symptoms such as gas and bloating, also known as a "die-off" reaction or Herxheimer reaction, as a result of gut bacteria changes.

## Handling Advice:

- Be Patient: Recognize that these symptoms are temporary and part of the gut microbiome's adjustment process.

- Reduce Dosage in the Short Term: Lower the supplement amount if symptoms are uncomfortable, then gradually raise it as your body adjusts.

While there are many advantages to using Vital Biome Gut Health 4-in-1 supplements, a more positive experience can be ensured by being aware of potential side effects and knowing how to manage them. As you begin, pay attention to how your body reacts, and seek medical advice as necessary.

# Chapter 9: FAQs on Vital Biome Gut Health 4-in-1 Supplements

This section answers some frequently asked questions (FAQs) about Vital Biome Gut Health 4-in-1 supplements, providing clarity and guidance on their use, benefits, and potential concerns.

1. What are Vital Biome Gut Health 4-in-1 Supplements?

**Answer:**

Vital Biome Gut Health 4-in-1 supplements promote digestive health by combining probiotics, prebiotics, digestive enzymes, and fiber in a single formulation. These components work together to maintain a healthy gut microbiome, improve digestion, increase nutrient absorption, and promote overall well-being.

2. Who Should Take These Supplements?

**Answer:**

These supplements are appropriate for adults who want to improve their digestive health, increase nutrient absorption, and boost immune function. They can be especially useful for people who are experiencing digestive discomfort, have irregular bowel movements, or want to maintain a healthy gut microbiome.

## 3. How Do I Use Vital Biome Gut Health 4-in-1 Supplements?

**Answer:**

Follow the dosage directions on the supplement label or as prescribed by your physician. Typically, these supplements are taken once or twice a day with meals. Starting with a lower dose and gradually increasing to the recommended amount will allow your body to adjust.

## 4. Are There Any Side Effects?

**Answer:**

When first taking the supplements, some people may experience mild side effects such as bloating, gas, or changes in bowel movements. These symptoms are usually temporary while your body adjusts. If the side effects persist or worsen, see a doctor.

## 5. Can I Take These Supplements with My Medication?

**Answer:**

While most supplements are safe, it's important to check with your doctor before starting any new one, especially if you're taking medication. Certain components may interact with medications, reducing their effectiveness or causing side effects.

## 6. What Is the Anticipated Duration Of The Outcomes?

**Answer:**

The time it takes to see results varies according to individual health conditions and lifestyle factors. Within a few weeks of consistent use, noticeable improvements in digestion and overall well-being can be observed. Patience and consistency are crucial.

## 7. Can I Use These Supplements if I Have Food Allergies?

**Answer:**

Check the ingredient list for possible allergens. If you have a history of allergies, consult a doctor before beginning the supplement. If you have an allergic reaction, stop using the product and seek medical attention.

## 8. Should I Refrigerate the Supplements?

**Answer:**

Storage instructions can vary depending on the formulation. Some probiotics must be refrigerated to maintain their potency, while others can be stored on the shelf. To ensure maximum efficacy, follow the storage guidelines on the product packaging.

## 9. What's The Difference Between Probiotics and Prebiotics?

**Answer:**

Probiotics are live beneficial bacteria that promote gut health, whereas prebiotics are nondigestible fibers that nourish these beneficial bacteria. Both are essential for a healthy gut microbiome and should be part of a well-balanced diet.

## 10. Can I Use These Supplements Long Term?

**Answer:**

Yes, Vital Biome Gut Health 4-in-1 supplements are intended for long-term use to maintain digestive health and overall well-being. Regular use can help keep the gut microbiome balanced and promote long-term health benefits.

Understanding the frequently asked questions about Vital Biome Gut Health 4-in-1 supplements allows you to make informed decisions and use them more effectively. By addressing common questions and concerns, we hope to provide clarity and support throughout your gut health journey.

# Conclusion: Embrace Your Journey to Optimal Gut Health.

Finally, it is crucial to consider the transforming journey that improved gut health can provide. The ideas and experience shared on these pages demonstrate how supporting your stomach can have a significant impact on your overall health. A healthy gut can alleviate stomach discomfort and increase your immune system, as well as improve mental clarity and energy levels.

The Vital Biome Gut Health 4-in-1 nutritional supplements provide a complete approach to promoting and maintaining gut health. These supplements address the intricacies of digestive health by mixing probiotics, prebiotics, digestive enzymes, and fiber. Scientific studies and real-life testimonials demonstrate the usefulness of these components, giving you confidence in the excellent results you can expect.

As you embark on your path to good gut health, remember that patience and consistency are essential. Each person's body is unique, and the time it takes to observe major changes may differ. Listen to your body, make adjustments as needed, and stay focused on your health goals.

It's also crucial to combine these supplements with a healthy diet, regular exercise, and a thoughtful lifestyle. Holistic health is more than just one component of well-being; it is the integration of numerous disciplines that benefit both your body and mind.

I hope that by sharing my personal story, you will be inspired and empowered to take care of your gut health. The journey to wellness is not always easy, but with the correct tools and information, it is possible.

Vital Biome Gut Health 4-in-1 nutritional supplements can be an important component of your health toolkit, helping you live a happier, healthier life.

Thank you for spending the time to read this book and invest in your health. May your road to greater gut health be fulfilling and transforming, guiding you to realize your full potential for well-being.

# Bonus: Exclusive Gut-Friendly Recipes

**Breakfast**

**1. Gut-Healing Smoothie**

- **Ingredients:**
    - One cup of unsweetened almond milk
    - One banana 1/2 cup frozen berries.
    - One spoonful of chia seeds
    - One spoonful of flaxseeds
    - half cup Greek yogurt (high in probiotics).
    - One teaspoon of honey (optional)
- **Instructions:**

    1. Fill a blender with all the ingredients.

    2. Blend until smooth.

    3. Pour the mixture into a glass and enjoy it.

**2. Overnight Oats with Probiotics:**

- **Ingredients:**
    - half cup of rolled oats
    - half a cup of unsweetened almond milk
    - one-quarter cup of Greek yogurt.

- One spoonful of chia seeds
- one teaspoon of honey
- half a teaspoon of cinnamon.
- Fresh berries for topping

- **Instructions:**

1. Combine chia seeds, honey, cinnamon, almond milk, Greek yogurt, and oats in a container.

2. Close and leave in the fridge for the entire night.

3. In the morning, garnish with fresh berries and serve.

**Lunch**

**3. Fermented Vegetable Salad:**

- **Ingredients:**
  - two cups mixed greens.
  - a half-cup of fermented vegetables (sauerkraut or kimchi)
  - half sliced avocado.
  - one-quarter cup of grated carrots
  - one-quarter cup of sliced cucumbers
  - one-quarter cup of half-cut cherry tomatoes
  - two tablespoons of olive oil
  - one tablespoon of apple cider vinegar.

- pepper and salt to taste.

- **Instructions:**

1. In a bowl, combine the mixed greens, avocado, fermented vegetables, carrots, cucumbers, and tomatoes.

2. Finish with a drizzle of olive oil and apple cider vinegar.

3. Add pepper and salt for seasoning, then serve.

## 4. Quinoa and Lentil Bowl

- **Ingredients:**
  - a half cup of cooked quinoa
  - a half cup of cooked lentils
  - one cup of steamed broccoli
  - one-quarter cup of sliced bell peppers
  - one-quarter cup of half-cut cherry tomatoes
  - Two teaspoons of tahini dressing

- **Instructions:**

1. Mix the quinoa, lentils, broccoli, bell peppers, and cherry tomatoes in a bowl.

2. Drizzle with tahini dressing and stir thoroughly.

3. Serve immediately.

**Dinner**

## 5. Gut-Friendly Chicken Stir-Fry:

- **Ingredients:**

  - one tablespoon of olive oil.

  - Two sliced chicken breasts

  - One cup of broccoli florets.

  - One sliced red bell pepper.

  - one sliced zucchini

  - Two minced garlic cloves

  - One tsp of ginger that has been freshly grated

  - two tablespoons of tamari (gluten-free soy sauce)

  - one tablespoon of apple cider vinegar

  - a tablespoon of honey.

- **Instructions:**

  1. Place the olive oil in a large saucepan and bring it to temperature over medium heat.

  2. Add the chicken and heat until it is brown.

  3. Stir-fry the broccoli, bell pepper, zucchini, ginger, and garlic for five to seven minutes.

  4. In a small bowl, combine the tamari, honey, and apple cider vinegar.

5. Pour the sauce over the stir fry and simmer for an additional 2 minutes.

6. Serve with brown rice or quinoa.


## 6. Salmon paired with asparagus and sauerkraut

- **Ingredients:**

  - 1 bunch of trimmed asparagus

  - 2 salmon fillets

  - 1 cup sauerkraut

  - A single tablespoon of olive oil.

  - Season with salt and pepper.

  - Serve with wedges of lemon.

- **Instructions:**

  1. Preheat the oven to 350 degrees Fahrenheit or 190 degrees Celsius.

  2. Place the salmon fillets on a baking sheet and sprinkle with pepper and salt.

  3. Put the asparagus in a circle around the salmon and drizzle with olive oil.

  4. Bake the fish for 15 to 20 minutes, or until it is cooked through.

5. Serve asparagus and salmon with lemon wedges and sauerkraut.

**Snacks**

## 7. Probiotic Yogurt Parfait

- **Ingredients:**

  - one cup of Greek yogurt.

  - a half cup of granola, ideally sugar-free.

  - 1/4 cup of berry mixture.

  - Include one tablespoon each of chia seeds and honey.

- **Instructions:**

  1. Put mixed berries, oats, and Greek yogurt in a glass.

  2. Sprinkle chia seeds on top and drizzle with honey.

  3. Serve right away.

## 8. Almond Butter and Apple Slices

- **Ingredients:**

  - One sliced apple

  - one tablespoon of chia seeds

- two tablespoons of almond butter.

- **Instructions:**

    1. Put the apple slices in a platter arrangement.

    2. Top each slice with almond butter.

    3. Sprinkle chia seeds over top and enjoy.


**Drinks**

## 9. Mocktail Kombucha

- **Ingredients:**

    - One cup of any flavor of kombucha

    - A single teaspoon of freshly squeezed lemon juice

    - half a cup of sparkling water.

    - Garnish with fresh mint leaves

- **Instructions:**

    1. Fill a glass with the kombucha, sparkling water, and lemon juice.

    2. Include ice and top with fresh mint leaves.

    3. Serve chilled.

## 10. Ginger Turmeric Tea:

- **Ingredients:**

  - two cups of water

  - 1 inch of freshly sliced ginger

  - one tablespoon of honey

  - one teaspoon of ground turmeric.

  - Slices of lemon to serve.

- **Instructions:**

  1. Pour boiling water into a pot.

  2. Add the ground turmeric and ginger slices and cook for ten minutes

  3. Pour the tea and strain it into a cup.

  4. Stir in the slices of lemon and honey.

  5. Enjoy while still warm.

# About The Author

Hazel Knight, a dedicated advocate for healthy lifestyle choices, makes her writing debut with **"Gut Health Revolution: The Benefits of Vital Biome Gut Health 4-in-1 Supplements for Men and Women."** With a background in nutrition and wellness coaching, Hazel is committed to assisting others in achieving optimal health through practical, science-based methods. Her dedication to encouraging gut health derives from her own transformative journey which inspired her to share tips and tactics for living a better life. Hazel's relatable style and evidence-based recommendations make her a trustworthy advisor on the path to wellness.

# Appreciation

*I would like to express my deepest gratitude to You for selecting my book, and I hope you enjoyed reading it. If you like it, would you please consider writing a review? Your feedback serve as motivation to me as an author and also makes the book more accessible to other readers. Thank you once again for your time and consideration. I hope that your journey towards wellness is filled with health and happiness.*